The Negative Calorie Diet:

60+ Life-changing Proven Recipes Helping You to Burn Body Fat, Lose Weight, and Boost Your Metabolism

[Second Edition]

processes, or directions contained within is the solitary and utter responsibility of the recipient reader. Under no circumstances will any legal responsibility or blame be held against the publisher for any reparation, damages, or monetary loss due to the information herein, either directly or indirectly.

Respective authors own all copyrights not held by the publisher.

The information herein is offered for informational purposes solely, and is universal as so. The presentation of the information is without contract or any type of guarantee assurance.

Table of Contents

Introduction

What comes into your mind when you read the word "diet"? I bet, for most people, diet means starvation or deprivation of food. Of course, this definition makes sense, right? If you want to lose weight, then going on a "diet" would mean skipping meals or cutting down your consumption of food.

Unfortunately, a lot of people would give up on their diets because they are not keen on the idea of going hungry; who wants to starve anyway? While others strive to follow their diet, even if it means going hungry, just to achieve the benefits of losing weight. However, what they don't know is that even though they're shedding pounds, their restricted diet might be limiting their bodies from the vitamins and other nutrients that it needs to function properly.

What if I told you that there's a diet that can help you burn fat, lose weight, and still encourage you to eat full meals and even snacks?

The Negative Calorie Diet is a meal program that encourages the dieters to eat meals. In fact, after a 10-day cleanse, a significant weight loss is expected. After that, you will enter a 20-day, eat all you can phase, which of course has meals that have negative calorie foods as ingredients. *I'll discuss more on that later.* But, the beauty of this diet is that you don't need to eliminate any type of food groups you can eat (however, junk food and processed foods are obviously eliminated), portions are not restricted, and you can eat until you're full, as long as you are eating negative calorie foods.

Since the negative calorie foods are whole foods that help the body burn fat, which in effect help you lose weight. These foods are also vitamin and mineral dense, so you are sure to get plenty of nutrients from your diet. Of course, when you follow a healthy diet, you also acquire the benefits of it such as—maintain a healthy weight, better blood sugar levels, and even reduce inflammation.

Before I go any further, let me thank you for purchasing this book. This book contains a brief introduction of the diet and a list of do's and don'ts as your guide. It is packed with 60 fat-burning recipes for breakfast, snacks, sides, smoothies, and main meals, which you can use for your meal plans.

Are you ready to eat and still burn fat? Turn to the first chapter now!

Chapter 1: A Brief Introduction of the Negative Calorie Diet

Eat and still burn fat? Yes, this may seem impossible to believe, but there are foods that you can consume that enables your body to shed fat even if you don't starve yourself to death. How is this possible you ask?

The foods that are included in the Negative Calorie Diet are foods (I will provide the list below) that are basically categorized as "thermogenic" foods. This means when you consume these foods, for example, broccoli, your body generates more heat as you digest it. It then revs up your metabolism making you burn calories as you eat; amazing right? What's even better is that these whole-foods provide you with quality calories and are packed with nutrients which supports your metabolism and over-all health; and they're satiating too so you can prevent those unnecessary bouts with hunger.

So a better understanding of negative calorie foods is that it isn't a food that doesn't contain calories, in fact, they do contain calories. However, when you consume them, your body expends more calories during digestion compared to the actual calories that the food contains.

Top 10 Negative Calorie Foods

1. **Green Leafy Vegetables** – Think of spinach, lettuce, kale, Swiss chard— these veggies that you hated so much as a child are rich in phytonutrients and are a good source of fiber. When you consume these vegetables, whether in your salad, smoothie, or omelet, you are actually helping your body to burn more calories as you consume them. What's even great is that these foods make you feel full for

longer periods of time, which can help you avoid unhealthy food cravings and overeating.

2. **Cruciferous Vegetables** – Some examples of this food are cauliflower, broccoli, and cabbage. Studies show that these vegetables contain a compound that controls the growth of fat cells. Like I said, there's no need for portion control in this diet so you can have as many of these vegetables as you like.

3. **Nightshades** – Eggplants, tomatoes, bell peppers, and chilies are examples of nightshades. There are three significant benefits that you can get from eating these vegetables, first off, they contain water, which makes you feel full when you consume them, they are rich in fiber which is great for digestion and managing your blood sugar levels, and finally, they contain the natural chemical, *capsaicin* that has a thermogenic effect in your body.

4. **Celery** – Like the other vegetables in this list, celery is also rich in fiber. Consuming this as snacks will make you feel satiated without the need of eating foods that are high in calories.

5. **Cucumber** – As a good source of insoluble fiber, cucumbers help in speeding up the movement of food in your digestive system and also limits your body's absorption of starch which help prevent blood sugar spikes.

6. **Berries** – These delicious tiny bombshells are considered as superfoods because they contain undeniable amounts of antioxidants and nutrients that are good for the body. Consuming berries can help burn-fat because of the thermogenic effect in your body, plus it also has compounds that regulate

a certain type of hormone that makes your brain believe that you're full.

7. **Citrus Fruits** – Coupled with exercise, citrus fruits, which is rich in Vitamin C, is seen to help burn as much as 30% more of fat during workouts. Some of the best examples of citrus fruits are: oranges, tangerines, grapefruit, and limes.

8. **Apples** – We all know the adage "An apple a day keeps the doctor away." However, did you know that eating apples can help you keep unwanted fats away? That's because this wonder fruit contains a compound called polyphenols that is proven to help reduce fat, especially in the belly area.

9. **Mushrooms** – Research show that this fungi contains molecules that helps bind cholesterol in your digestive system, preventing it to enter into your system. Mushrooms are a great ingredient to your meals, especially if your goal is to lose weight.

10. **Almonds** – Consuming just a handful of this protein and fiber-rich nut is seen to help keep you satiated throughout the day. This means you will have lesser hunger pangs and will help you only eat what you need (and not want) because you already feel full.

The design of the Negative Calorie Diet requires dieters to undergo a 10-Day Cleanse to clear your system with toxins and chemicals that affect your body's metabolism. During this phase you can consume as much as four detox drinks or smoothies made of negative calorie foods and one meal like a salad or soup using the ingredients listed above.

After this detox phase you will then have a 20-Day Eat-All-You-Can phase that also includes the ingredients above plus added good source of protein. Obviously, what you want to choose are lean cuts of protein, which are also considered as thermogenic foods. Research shows that increasing the consumption of lean proteins to 30% in your diet can actually help you lose that stubborn belly fat.

Good Sources of Protein

1. **Lean cuts of beef, as well as lean ground beef**

2. **Free-range chicken and organic eggs**

3. **Turkey**

4. **Tuna, preferably wild-caught**

5. **Mussels**

6. **Shrimp**

7. **Clams**

8. **Crabmeat**

Do's and Don'ts

o **Don't Skip Meals** – Never skip any meals, yes, breakfast included. Make sure you eat three main meals and a snack every day. This is because skipping meals will make you tend to overeat and be unconscious of the foods you choose to consume. By eating meals every 3-4 hours, you make sure that your metabolism is also working and doing its job all day.

- **Choose Whole Foods** – Always choose foods that have not been processed or refined. This means that you have to stay away from ready-to-eat meals, junk food, non-organic, GMO food, and other foods that have artificial additives (soda, artificial sweeteners, etc.) on them. Some of the best examples of whole foods are fruits and vegetables, nuts, eggs, poultry and fish.

  While this diet does not eliminate the consumption of macronutrients (fat, protein, and carbs) it is recommended that you limit dairy and refined carbohydrates in your meals.

- **Shop in local markets** – A great place to find fresh and organic produce is in local markets. This way, you can literally have ingredients for your meals straight from the farm to your plate; which is ideal in a healthy diet.

- **Increase your intake of water** – Water is the *true* negative calorie food. Make sure you drink not less than eight glasses of water every day to increase your metabolism.

- **Spend more time in the kitchen** – Of course, to make sure that you're only eating healthy foods with negative calorie recipes, it'll be ideal that you prepare your meals yourself, this means you have to spend more time in the kitchen.

  If you want to lose weight and change your lifestyle, you must be ready to make some sacrifices and adjustments such as making your own meals.

- o **Never be afraid to try new recipes** – I have provided you with 60 recipes in this book that you can cook while on the diet. Use these recipes for your meals, but also never be afraid to make recipes of your own. Just make sure that the first 10 days of the diet will only be limited on the top 10 negative calorie foods and then on the 20-day phase, you can add or substitute the ingredients you like in the recipes, for example, substituting chicken to turkey.

- o **Create a Meal Plan** – In order to lose weight, you have to strictly stick to the diet for 30 straight days. To help make things easier for you, you need to create your own meal plan to guide you in the diet. I hope that you use the recipes found in this book to create yours. Mix and match the recipes and enjoy eating them.

Chapter 2: Fat-Burning Breakfast Recipes

Waffles and Berries

This is a low-cal, guilt-free waffle recipe you and the whole family will surely love!

Ingredients

4 whole-grain waffle
¼ cup blueberries, frozen
¼ cup raspberries, frozen
2 tbsp. pecan nuts, roughly chopped
4 tsp. maple syrup

Procedure

1. Combine the blueberries, raspberries, and maple syrup in a bowl and place in the microwave to thaw for 3 minutes.

2. Place the waffles on an oven and lightly toast for a few minutes. Serve with the mixed berries, and chopped pecans on top.

Serves: 2

Calories: 41 per serving

The Perfect Bowl of Apple n' Oats

Enjoy this hearty and easy-to-make bowl of breakfast that can fill you up before you start the daily grind.

Ingredients

2 pcs. large apples, diced
4 tbsp. oat bran
1 cup vanilla almond milk, unsweetened
½ tsp. cinnamon, ground
½ tsp. coconut oil
1 tbsp. toasted almond, chopped
1 tsp. stevia

Procedure

3. Heat a non-stick skillet over medium fire and melt the coconut oil in it. Throw in the apples to the pan, add the cinnamon and cook for about 3 minutes, or until the apples soften.

4. Turn of the heat and pour the almond milk, oat bran, and stevia. Stir well.

5. Turn on the fire again on medium heat and stir. Allow to simmer for about a minute, or until the mixture thickens.

6. Transfer into two bowls and garnish with the chopped almonds on top.

Serves: 2

Calories: 137 per serving

Omelet and Toast

If you're looking for a "heavier" breakfast to fill your belly on a busy morning, then this complete breakfast plate is what you will need to whip up in your kitchen.

Ingredients

2 slices whole-grain toast
1 tsp. almond butter
2 whole organic or free-range eggs
4 eggs whites, organic or free range
4 slices turkey bacon, cooked and chopped
2 cups spinach, chopped
1 tsp. olive oil

Procedure

1. In a medium-sized bowl, stir the eggs, spinach, and bacon together. Whisk well.

2. Heat the olive oil on a non-stick skillet over medium fire and pour the egg mixture.

3. Cook until the egg sets.

4. Serve with toasted whole wheat with almond butter spread.

Serves: 2

Calories: 308 per serving

Sunrise Toast

Ever tried avocado and egg on your toast? Try this creamy and delish toast recipe for breakfast and even during snack time.

Ingredients

½ Haas avocado
2 pcs. free-range eggs, poached
2 slices gluten-free or whole wheat bread, toasted
2 slices of tom
4 cups baby spinach
Celtic salt
Black pepper, ground
Sriracha sauce (optional)

Procedure

1. Place a skillet over medium-high fire. When the pan is hot, throw in the spinach, and cook for a few minutes, or until wilted.

2. Put the cooked spinach on a colander and press out the remaining water from the spinach and then transfer to a large bowl.

3. Season the spinach with salt, pepper and Sriracha sauce (add as much as you want).

4. Meanwhile, mash the avocado in a small bowl using a fork and season with salt.

5. Lay the toast slices two plates and spread the avocado mash on top of each bread slice. Top with the tomato slice, follow by the wilted spinach and then finally, with the poached eggs.

Serves: 2

Calories: 180 per serving

Tomato and Cheese

Don't you just love the perfect combination of cheese and tomatoes? Here's a simple open face sandwich perfect for people who are on the rush.

Ingredients

2 pcs. whole-wheat bagel
4 thick slices of tomato
4 tbsp. cream cheese, low fat
Celtic salt and freshly ground pepper to taste

Procedure

1. Cut the bagels in half and place in the oven to toast.

2. Generously spread the cream cheese on the bagel slices and top with tomato slices.

3. Season with salt and pepper. Serve.

Serves: 2

Calories: 302 per serving

Mixed Berries and Quinoa

A perfect breakfast to consume after your morning workout. This mixed-berry bowl will provide you the energy you need for the day and will surely help you burn more fats.

Ingredients

¼ cup strawberries, sliced
¼ cup blueberries
¼ raspberries
¼ cup blackberries
4 tbsp. cooked quinoa
½ cup toasted almonds, chopped
2 tbsp. Greek yogurt, fat-free

Procedure

1. Mix the berries in equal amounts into two serving bowls.

2. In a separate, combine the quinoa and toasted almonds. Stir well.

3. Top the mixed berries with the quinoa mixture and scoop a tablespoon of yogurt on top of each bowl.

4. Serve.

Serves: 2

Calories: 142 per serving

Mushroom and Kale Omelet

Get a great load of nutrients such as Vitamin A, C, calcium, iron, and fiber with this healthy low-calorie omelet.

Ingredients

6 egg whites

2 cups portabella mushrooms, sliced
2 cups kale leaves, ribs removed and chopped
1 tbsp. shallots, chopped fine
Celtic salt to taste
1/8 tsp. red pepper flakes
1 tsp. olive oil
1 tbsp. Parmigiano Reggiano, grated (optional)

Procedure

1. Set oven at 350F.

2. In a bowl, whisk the egg whites using an electronic mixer until it turns foamy. Set aside.

3. Meanwhile, heat the olive oil in an oven-safe pan over medium fire. Add the mushrooms to the pan and allow to cook until it softens.

4. Season the mushrooms with salt and then transfer on a plate. Set aside.

5. Using the same pan, throw in the shallots and red pepper flakes and cook for 2 minutes. Place the kale in the pan. Stir and cook for 4 minutes, or until the kale is wilted.

6. Place the cooked mushrooms in the pan with the kale along with the foamy egg whites. Allow egg to cook for a few minutes until it is about to set.

7. Turn of the heat and place the pan in the oven to cook for 2 minutes.

8. Take out the oven and fold the egg to make an omelet.

9. Divide the omelet into 2 servings.

Serves: 2

Calories: 108 per serving

Breakfast Frittata

This recipe is an all-in-one breakfast that will give you a surge of energy that you need while also helping you burn fat. Plus, this frittata is also a great way to encourage your children to eat their veggies.

Ingredients

6 egg whites
4 cups baby spinach, washed and roughly chopped
1 tbsp. water

½ cup fresh basil leaves, chopped
1 tsp. garlic, minced
½ cup red onion, sliced thin
½ cup grape tomatoes, sliced in half
A pinch of crushed red pepper flakes
Celtic salt to taste
1 tsp. olive oil

Procedure

1. Set the oven at 350F.

2. Put the chopped spinach with 1 tbsp. of water in a microwave-safe bowl and cover with parchment paper. Place in the microwave and cook on high for 4-5 minutes.

3. Press the spinach and drain the excess water. Set aside.

4. In another bowl, whisk the egg whites using an electronic beater until foamy. Set aside.

5. Heat the olive oil in a huge non-stick pan over medium-high fire. Sauté the garlic for about a minute and then add the red pepper flakes, onion and chopped basil leaves.

6. Lower the heat to medium, stir the vegetables, and cook for 3 minutes.

7. Add the grape tomatoes and baby spinach to the pan and also pour the egg whites. Stir well.

8. Turn of the heat when the eggs are about to set.

9. Transfer the pan in the oven to cook for about 2 minutes, or until the eggs are thoroughly cooked.

10. Serve hot.

Serves: 2

Calories: 147 per serving

Asparagus, Poached Eggs, and Toast

As simple as this dish may seem, this recipe is packed with quality calories and provide you with a good amount of calcium.

Ingredients

4 slices whole-wheat bread
4 free-range eggs, poached
(simmer for 6 minutes to poach)
½ lb. asparagus, trimmed
2 tbsp. parmesan cheese, grated
Celtic salt and pepper to taste
1 tbsp. olive oil

Procedure

1. Lay the bread slices and asparagus on a baking sheet. Drizzle with the olive oil and season with salt and pepper. Toss the asparagus using your hands.

2. Place in a broiler set on high temperature and toast the bread for about 2 minutes each side.

3. Remove the bread from the broiler when toasted. Toss the asparagus and continue to broil for 5-8 minutes more.

4. Divide the toast on 2 serving plates and top with the broiled asparagus. Finally, place the poached eggs on top and sprinkle with grated parmesan cheese.

Serves: 2

Calories: 310 per serving

Refreshing Bowl of Breakfast

A great mix of negative calorie foods, this bowl of salad will help your body burn fat and also has properties that flushes toxins out of your body.

Ingredients

2 cups tangerines, cut into bite-sized pieces
1 cup grape fruit, cut into bite-sized pieces
1 large cucumber, sliced
¼ cup fresh basil leaves, chopped

Procedure

1. Combine all the ingredients into two separate serving bowls.

2. Serve immediately

Serves: 2

Calories: 134 per serving

Avocado Pizza Breakfast

Pizza for breakfast? Definitely! Check out this recipe for a healthy "pizza" breakfast meal.

Ingredients

2 whole-grain tortillas
1 ripe avocado, pitted and peeled
2 organic eggs
2 tsp. olive oil
1 tsp. fresh lemon juice
salt and pepper to taste

Procedure

1. Warm the tortillas in an oven for 30 seconds.

2. Meanwhile, place the avocado meat and lemon juice in a bowl. Season with salt and pepper and mash well using a fork to achieve a smooth consistency.

3. Scoop the avocado mixture and spread over the tortillas.

4. Heat the olive oil on a non-stick pan over medium heat and cook the eggs, sunny-side up style. Cook until the egg yoks are just about to thicken.

5. Place eggs on top of the "pizza". Season with salt and pepper.

6. Serve warm.

Serves: 2

Calories: 299 per serving

Zesty Salmon Cakes

A recipe you can make ahead and then freeze when you're not ready to eat yet.

Ingredients

18 oz. salmon chunks
½ cup scallions
½ cup olives, pitted
2 tbsp. fresh dill, coarsely chopped
1 tbsp. fresh thyme
1 tsp. lemon zest
salt and pepper to taste
1 tbsp. olive oil

Procedure

1. Place the scallions, olives, dill, and thyme in a food processor and blend until the mixture is finely chopped. Transfer into a bowl, season with salt and pepper, and mix in the lemon zest.

2. Slowly add the salmon chunks into the food processor and pulse for a few times to chop.

3. Add the salmon into the bowl with chopped scallions and mix well.

4. Using your hands, create 6-8 pcs. of patties. Place in the fridge to chill for at least 20 minutes.

5. Drizzle the olive oil on a non-stick pan over medium fire. Cook the salmon cakes for 4 minutes on each side or until it is cooked through.

6. Serve with lemon wedges on the side.

Serves: 4 (2 cakes each)

Calories: 214 per serving

Make Ahead Slow-Cooked Oats

This is another recipe you can make at night and enjoy for breakfast at the morning.

Ingredients

4 cups water
1 cup steel-cut oats
¼ cup dried apricots, chopped
¼ cup dried cranberries
salt to taste

Procedure

1. Combine the water, oats, apricots, cranberries, and salt in a slow cooker set on low.

2. Cover the slow cooker and cook for 8 hours.

Serves: 4

Calories: 193 per serving

Granola Pumpkin Spice

No-sweat breakfast recipe to get you going in the morning.

Ingredients

1 can pumpkin, mashed
2 pcs. whole-grain granola, crumbled
4 tsp. raw honey
12 oz. low-fat yogurt
½ tsp. pumpkin-pie spice

Procedure

1. Combine the low-fat yogurt, honey, and pumpkin-pie spice.

2. To serve, layer the pumpkin mash, granola, and yogurt mixture in a parfait glass.

Serves: 2

Calories: 304 per serving

Morning Dessert

Dessert in the morning? *Why not!*

Ingredients

1 cup non-fat yogurt, peach flavor
1 cup fresh raspberries
1 cup frozen pineapple chunks
2 tsp. granola

Procedure

1. Layer the yogurt and raspberries in a glass. Sprinkle with granola on top.

Serves: 2

Calories: 109 per serving

Monkey Bites

Love bananas for breakfast? This recipe gives you another reason to go bananas in the morning!

Ingredients

1 ripe banana, sliced
2 tbsp. almond butter
1 tsp. raw honey
1 whole-wheat bagel, cut in half

Procedure

1. In a small bowl, combine the almond butter and honey.

2. Place the bagel halves in an oven and toast.

3. Spread the almond butter mixture over the bagels and top with banana slices.

Serves: 1

Calories: 284 per serving

Chapter 3: All-You-Can-Eat Snacks, Smoothies, and Sides

Snacks
Celery-Peanut Butter Sticks

Looking for healthy snacks that your kids will also love? Try this easy to make snack made with negative calorie food and is also rich in protein.

Ingredients

6 pcs. celery stalks
4 tbsp. all-natural peanut butter
2 tbsp. raisins, or dried cranberries

Procedure

1. Lay the celery sticks on a serving plate and generously spread the peanut butter on top.

2. Top with raisins or cranberries.

Serves: 2 (3 sticks per person)

Calories: 72 per serving

Candied Bell Peppers

Warning! You'll surely can't stop munching on these delish bites!

Ingredients

1 red bell pepper
1 yellow bell pepper
1 tbsp. maple syrup
Procedure

1. Set the oven at 150F.

2. Cut the bell peppers in half and remove the core and seeds. Slice them into half an inch strips and transfer in a bowl.

3. Drizzle the bell peppers with maple syrup and toss using your hands.

4. Cover a baking sheet with parchment paper and lay the bell pepper strips on it. Make sure that the bell pepper are separated from each other.

5. Place the bell pepper to cook in the oven with the door open for about 5 inches and cook for 8 hours to allow the bell pepper to dehydrate. (You can also use a dehydrator to do this so you can skip #1 and #5).

6. You can store these candies in an air tight container.

Serves: 6

Calories: 12 per serving (5 strips of candy)

Roasted Veggie Salad

A hearty and healthy salad made with an alternative dressing for artificial store-brought salad dressing.

Ingredients

¼ cup balsamic vinegar
½ cup non-fat yogurt
1 tbsp. extra virgin olive oil
1 tbsp. flat leaf parsley, chopped
1 tsp. garlic, minced
¼ cup roasted bell pepper, diced
1 eggplant, sliced thick
2 pcs. cucumber, sliced thick
1 small white onion, sliced thick

Procedure

1. Place a saucepan over medium heat and pour balsamic vinegar. Let it simmer for 3-4 minutes to allow it to reduce. Transfer in a small bowl, set aside to cool.

2. When the balsamic vinegar is at room temperature, combine it with the yogurt, extra virgin olive oil, parsley, and minced garlic. Whisk well.

3. Lay the sliced vegetables on baking sheet and drizzle with half of the balsamic and yogurt mixture. Toss gently to coat.

4. Heat your grill and roast the vegetables for about 4 minutes.

5. Transfer the roasted veggies on a serving plate and sprinkle with diced bell peppers. And drizzle with the remaining vinaigrette. Toss again and serve.

Serves: 2

Calories: 180 per serving

Easy Kale Side Dish

Packed with Vitamin C, beta-carotene, calcium, and potassium, this super-easy to make side dish is a perfect pair for any lean meat meals.

Ingredients

1 lb. kale, ribs removed and chopped
1 tsp. olive oil
1 tsp. garlic, chopped
1 cup black-eyed peas, drained
½ tsp. apple cider vinegar
¼ tsp. red pepper flakes

Procedure

1. Pour water into a pot (about ¼ full) and bring to a boil. Throw in the kale to the pot and cover. Cook the leaves for about 15 minutes while stirring occasionally.

2. Drain the kale and set aside. (You can keep the water from this as a vegetable stock)

3. Meanwhile, place a non-stick pan over medium-low fire and drizzle with olive oil. Sauté the garlic for 2 minutes and then add the black-eyed peas to the pan. Stir for a minute and then add the red pepper flakes and cook for 2 minutes more.

4. Lower the heat and then add the boiled kale leaves.

5. Turn off the heat and place on a serving plate. Drizzle with apple cider when you're about to serve.

6. Serve warm.

Serves: 3

Calories: 120 per serving

Apple, Cheese, and Nuts Salad

Sweet, salty, and crunchy— everything you like in a salad!

Ingredients

2 Pink Lady apples
¼ cup pistachio, roughly chopped
3 tbsp. feta cheese, crumbled
½ cup non-fat yogurt
½ juice of lime
a pinch of black pepper
a pinch of cayenne pepper

Procedure

1. In a salad bowl, whisk the cayenne and black pepper with the yogurt.

2. Add the apples and juice of lime into the bowl and toss well.

3. Place in the fridge for at least an hour to chill.

4. Before serving, add the crumbled feta on top with the chopped pistachios.

Serves: 2

Calories: 200 per serving

Broccoli Salad to Go

Want to bring snacks or light lunch to work? Here's a perfect salad recipe for that!

Ingredients

½ cup broccoli florets, chopped
½ cup boiled chicken, cubed
1 celery stalk, sliced thin
½ cup carrot, diced
4 tbsp. dried cranberries
4 tbsp. onion, chopped
2 tsp. sunflower seeds
¼ cup non-fat yogurt
½ tbsp. honey
½ tsp. vinegar

Procedure

1. In a salad bowl, combine the broccoli, chicken cubes, celery, carrots, cranberries, and onion.

2. In a smaller bowl, combine the yogurt, honey, and vinegar.

3. Mix the salad dressing with the vegetables and sprinkle with sunflower seeds.

4. Serve.

Serves: 2 (2/3 cup per serving)

Calories: 110 per serving

Zesty Kale Salad

Can't get enough of kale? Here's a refreshing salad recipe that stars you favorite green leafy veg.

Ingredients

5 cups kale, stemmed and sliced thin
¼ cup toasted walnuts, chopped
4 tbsp. pitted olives, chopped
2 tsp. capers, rinsed and finely chopped
1 clove of garlic, minced
4 tbsp. extra virgin olive oil
1 tbsp. fresh lemon juice
½ tsp. dried oregano
salt and pepper to taste

Procedure

1. Whisk the olive oil, garlic, lemon juice, oregano, salt and pepper in a salad bowl.

2. Add the kale, walnuts, olives, and capers to the bowl. Toss well to coat with the dressing.

3. Serve immediately.

Serves: 4

Calories: 166 per serving

No-Bake Homemade Oat Bars

Here's a treat that you can store in your pantry so you will always have something you can eat during snack time.

Ingredients

½ cup old fashioned oats
2 cups apple chips, freeze dried
¼ cup dried cranberries
¼ cup slivered almonds, toasted
2 tbsp. almond butter
3 tbsp. honey
a pinch of Celtic salt
a pinch of cayenne pepper

Procedure

1. Mix the apple chips, cranberries, almonds, and oats in a large bowl.

2. In a separate bowl, mix the almond butter, honey, salt, and cayenne. Combine well.

3. Pour the honey mixture to the large bowl and stir well. Make sure everything is well coated.

4. Cover a baking sheet with a cling wrap and transfer the oat mixture in the middle of the cling wrap.

5. Fold the cling wrap over the mixture and make it into a shape of a bar.

6. Cut this huge bar into 4-5 smaller bars.

7. You can store these bars in the fridge or in an airtight jar for 5 days.

Serves: Makes 4-5 bars

Calories: 211 per serving

Chicken on Lettuce Cups

Enjoy this low-cal, flavorful snack on a lazy Sunday afternoon!

Ingredients
8 oz. lean ground chicken
1 green onion, diced
1 clove of garlic, minced
¼ cup white onion, diced
½ tbsp. jalapeno, minced
2 tbsp. fresh lime juice
1 tsp. coconut aminos
½ head of iceberg lettuce,
-separate leaves to create cups
½ cup cilantro, chopped
salt and pepper to taste
1 and ½ tbsp. olive oil

Procedure

1. Heat 1 tbsp. olive oil on a non-stick pan over high temperature. When the oil is hot, add the ground chicken, and cook until brown for 3-4 minutes.

2. Move the cooked chicken to one side of the pan and then add the remaining olive oil to the pan. Sauté the garlic, white and green onions, and jalapeno to the pan and stir for 30 seconds.

3. Combine all the ingredients and then drizzle with lime juice and coconut aminos. Season with salt and pepper.

4. Serve the cooked chicken on top of the lettuce cups. Serve warm.

Serves: 3-4

Calories:120 per serving

Cobb Salad

Enjoy this classic salad recipe for your healthy snacks. (Skip the bacon, of course!)

Ingredients
1 cooked chicken breast fillet, cut into cubes
1 head romaine lettuce, chopped
1 ripe avocado, pitted, peeled, cut into cubes
1 cup grape tomato, sliced
2 hard-boiled eggs, sliced

For the dressing:
¼ cup extra virgin olive oil
4 tbsp. red wine vinegar
½ tsp. maple syrup
salt and pepper to taste

Procedure

1. Whisk the salad dressing in a large bowl. Mix well.

2. Add the salad ingredients with the dressing and toss well. Make sure to coat the veggies and chicken with the dressing for a flavorful salad.

Serves: 3

Calories:282 per serving

Strawberries and Chocolates

Feeling a little fancy this afternoon? Here's a strawberry and chocolate snack recipe that won't hurt your diet.

Ingredients

8 medium-sized strawberries
4 tbsp. toasted almonds, chopped
½ cup dark chocolate, no-sugar added

Procedure

1. Place the dark chocolate in a microwave oven safe bowl and place in the microwave to melt on high temperature for about 30 seconds or more. Make sure that you watch out for the chocolate so you won't burn it. You can take it out of the microwave as soon as you see the whole chocolate is almost melted.

2. Take the strawberries and carefully dip it in the chocolate on piece at a time. And then roll over the chopped almonds.

3. Place in a plate with a parchment paper on top and place in the fridge to chill before serving.

Serves: 2 (4 strawberries per serving)

Calories: 131 per serving

Mixed Berries and Homemade Cream

Who doesn't love berries and cream? This is a no-sweat recipe you can make for yourself and the whole family on a lazy weekend.

Ingredients

2 cup mixed berries, your choice of blueberries, strawberries, raspberries, etc.
1 orange, cut into bite-size chunks
4 tbsp. Greek yogurt, non-fat
½ cup vanilla almond milk, unsweetened
(separate ½ tbsp. milk)
1 tsp. clear gelatin powder
3 tbsp. agave nectar or honey
1 vanilla bean, cut in half

Procedure

1. Mix the gelatin with ½ tbsp. almond milk in a small bowl and set aside.

2. Whisk the remaining almond milk and agave nectar in a sauce pan heated over medium-low fire.

3. Bring into a simmer and scrape the vanilla beans into the milk mixture.

4. Pour the gelatin mixture into the pot and whisk well.

5. Transfer the almond milk mixture in a steel bowl and combine with the Greek yogurt.

6. Place this bowl in a larger bowl half-filled with ice and water. While the bowl is soaked in the ice bath,

whip the almond milk mixture using a handheld mixer until you achieve a thick cream.

7. Divide the mixed berries into two separate serving bowls and top with your homemade cream.

Serves: 2

Calories: 128 per serving

Soups
Savory Mushroom Soup

Fill your belly with this warm and savory mushroom soup.

Ingredients

9 cups mushrooms, sliced
1 medium carrot, diced
2 tsp. olive oil
1 tsp garlic, minced
½ cup scallions, sliced thin
1 ½ cup homemade vegetable broth
1 cup water
1 ½ cup non-fat milk
¼ tsp. dried thyme
pepper to taste

Procedure

1. Drizzle the olive oil in a large sauce pan over medium-high temperature.

2. Sauté the garlic and onions for about a minute and then add the thyme and a dash of pepper. Cook for another 3 minutes.

3. Add the sliced mushrooms, vegetable broth, water, and bring to a boil.

4. Remove the half of the vegetables from the pot and set aside.

5. Transfer the remaining vegetables and soup from the pot in a blender and mix until smooth. Gradually add the non-fat milk to the mixture and blend again.

6. Place both the pureed vegetables and the other half that you set aside in a sauce pan and allow to simmer again on medium-low heat for 5 minutes.

7. Serve hot.

Serves: 4

Calories: 120 per serving

Fat-Burning Chili Soup

Are you looking for something spicy to help burn your fat? Try this flavor-packed soup recipe today!

Ingredients

½ lb. chicken breast fillet, cut in cubes
1 yellow bell pepper, diced
1 carrot, sliced
3 tbsp. chili powder

1 cup kidney beans
1 can all natural-diced tomatoes, no-salt added
1 can low sodium beef broth
1 tbsp. olive oil
½ tbsp. garlic, minced
½ cup onion, chopped
salt and pepper to taste

Procedure

1. Drizzle olive oil in a large sauce pan heat over medium fire. Place the chicken cubes and cook until the chicken turns brown. Set aside.

2. Using the same pot, sauté the garlic with the onion and bell pepper for about a minute and then add the carrots. Cook and stir for about 4-5 minutes.

3. Add the chili powder to the pot and cook again for 2 minutes.

4. Then add the kidney beans, canned diced tomatoes (with liquid), beef broth, and chicken in the pot. Allow to simmer for 12-15 minutes or until the vegetables are tender.

5. Season with salt and pepper. Serve hot.

Serves: 4

Calories: 200 per serving

Roasted Veggie Soup

Enjoy a bowl of this delicious asparagus and cauliflower medley!

Ingredients

4 cups cauliflower florets, chopped
1 bunch asparagus, trimmed
2 cups vegetable broth
¼ tsp. garlic powder
¼ tsp. onion powder
pinch of cayenne
salt and pepper to taste

Procedure

1. Set oven at 400F.

2. Lay the cauliflower florets and asparagus on a baking sheet and place in the oven to cook for 20 minutes, or until the asparagus is tender.

3. Pour the vegetable broth in a pot and add the roasted vegetables. Bring to a simmer and cook for about 10 minutes.

4. Transfer the mixture into a blender, add the garlic and onion powder, cayenne, salt and pepper. Blend until you achieve a smooth consistency.

5. Serve warm.

Serves: 2-3

Calories: 78 per serving

Mixed Vegetable Stew

A simple recipe for a vegetable soup packed with negative calorie ingredients.

Ingredients

3 cups vegetable stock
½ cup celery, diced
1 cup cabbage, shredded
1 cup baby spinach
1 cup zucchini, diced
½ cauliflower florets, chopped
½ cup green beans, cut into bite-sized pieces
½ cup turnip, diced
2 cloves of garlic, minced
1 small onion, diced
1 pc. jalapeno chili, seeded, chopped
salt and pepper to taste

Procedure

1. Place all the ingredients (except the spinach) in a large pot and bring to a boil.

2. Reduce the heat to a simmer and continue cooking for 20 minutes. Season with salt and pepper.

3. Add the spinach and cook for a minute.

4. Serve warm.

Serves: 3

Calories: 66 per serving

Chicken and Spinach Soup

An Italian inspired recipe that is a good source of protein and fiber.

Ingredients

4 oz. chicken breast fillet, cut into chunks
3 cups baby spinach, chopped
1 small can beans, rinsed and drained
1 tbsp. olive oil (divided)
¼ cup carrot, diced
¼ cup bell pepper diced
1 clove of garlic, minced
3 cups low-sodium chicken stock
1 tsp. marjoram, dried
4 tbsp. Parmesan cheese, grated
3 tsp. fresh basil leaves, chopped
salt and pepper to taste

Procedure

1. Heat ½ tbsp. of olive oil in a saucepan. Throw in the bell pepper and carrots and sauté for a minute. Add the chicken and cook for about 4-5 minutes or until the chicken is lightly brown.

2. Add the minced garlic and stir for a minute.

3. Add the chicken stock and marjoram. Set the heat to high and bring to a boil.

4. Reduce the heat and simmer for 5 minutes. Stir occasionally.

5. Take out the chicken cubes from the pot and set aside.

6. Add the baby spinach and beans and then cook for another 5 minutes.

7. In a food processor, pulse the basil leaves, parmesan cheese, and the remaining olive oil. Blend until you achieve a paste-like consistency.

8. Add the pesto paste into the pot and then put back the chicken.

9. Season with salt and pepper and serve hot.

Serves: 2-3

Calories: 204 per serving

Fragrant Fish Poached Soup

Try this delicate soup recipe to warm your hungry belly.

Ingredients

4 cups low-sodium vegetable broth
16 oz. tilapia fillets, cut in chunks
1 bunch arugula, trimmed and chopped
1 cup carrots, finely chopped
¼ cup fresh mint leaves, sliced thin
2 scallions, finely chopped
1 lemon, zested and juiced
2 cups water

Procedure

1. Place the vegetable broth in a large pot and heat over medium-high fire. Add the lemon juice and zest and stir well.

2. Reduce the heat to medium or low and add the tilapia fillets. Cook for 5 minutes or until the fish is tender.

3. Divide the soup into 4 different serving bowls and garnish with arugula, carrots, and mint leaves.

4. Serve hot.

Serves: 4

Calories: 239 per serving

Viet-Inspired Beef Soup

Have a taste of Vietnam in your own home with this recipe!

Ingredients

8 oz. lean cut of beef, cut into chunks
1 tsp. olive oil
2 cups bok choy, chopped
2 cups low-sodium, chicken stock
1 cup water
2 oz. rice noodles
1 tsp. tamari
1 cup mung bean sprouts
2 tbsp. basil, chopped

Procedure

1. Drizzle the olive oil in a large pot. Add the beef and stir for about 2 minutes. Remove the beef from the pot and set aside.

2. Add the chopped bok choy to the pot and cook for 2 minutes or until the leaves start to wilt.

3. Pour the stock and water. Cover the pot and bring to a boil.

4. Add the rice noodles, tamari, and allow to simmer for 5 minutes.

5. Bring the beef back to the pot and cook for another 2 minutes.

6. Serve the soup into 2-3 serving bowls and garnish with mung bean sprouts and chopped basil leaves.

Serves: 3-4

Calories: 235 per serving

Smoothies
Combo Negative Calorie Food Shake

All the citrus and fat-burning goodness in one cup!

Ingredients

1 cup spinach
1 pc. orange, peel and seeds removed
½ banana, frozen
½ cup pomegranate juice
ice cubes

Procedure

1. Combine all the ingredients in a blender and mix until you achieve a smooth consistency.

Serves: 1

Calories: 200 per serving

Kale and Orange Smoothie

A refreshing smoothie that is rich in protein and will fill you up for a busy afternoon.

Ingredients

1 cup kale, ribs removed and chopped
1 orange, peeled and seeds removed
2 tbsp. protein powder, vanilla flavor
1 cup water
1/8 tsp. cinnamon powder
1/8 tsp. ginger powder

Procedure

1. Combine all the ingredients in a blender and mix until you achieve a smooth consistency.

Serves: 1

Calories: 300 per serving

Green Detox Shake

This recipe is a perfect drink during the 10-day phase of the Negative Calorie Diet

Ingredients

1 cup kale or spinach, chopped
1 cup cilantro
1 cup zucchini, chopped
½ Haas avocado
1 cup pineapple chunks
1 cup green tea, chilled
4 tbsp. juice of lemon
1 tbsp. grated ginger

Procedure

1. Combine all the ingredients in a blender and mix until you achieve a smooth consistency.

Serves: 1

Calories: 270 per serving

Peaches and Greens Smoothie

A great drink to chug down loads of greens and fruits.

Ingredients

2 cups baby spinach
2 tbsp. protein powder, vanilla flavor
1 cup almond milk, unsweetened
1 cup peaches, frozen
½ cup pineapple chunks
½ banana, frozen
1 tbsp. flax seed

Procedure

1. Combine all the ingredients in a blender and mix until you achieve a smooth consistency.

Serves: 1

Calories: 436 per serving

Sunshine Shake

Grab this delicious fruit and vegetable shake to brighten up your morning.

Ingredients

2 cups frozen peach, sliced
1 cup fresh orange juice
1 cup fresh carrot juice
1 tbsp. ginger, chopped
2 tbsp. flax seed, ground

Procedure

1. Combine all the ingredients in a blender and mix until you achieve a smooth consistency.

Serves: 1

Calories: 209 per serving

Berry-licious Smoothie

High-fiber, low-calorie, and gluten-free shake—what more can you ask for?

Ingredients

½ cup blueberries
½ cup raspberries
½ cup cranberries
½ cup strawberries,
1 frozen banana
1 cup pomegranate juice
½ cup water

Procedure

1. Combine all the ingredients in a blender and mix until you achieve a smooth consistency.

Serves: 2-3

Calories: 206 per serving

Green Pineapple Shake

Loads of negative calorie ingredients in one glass!

Ingredients

½ cup pineapple, chunked

1 pc. frozen banana
½ cup ripe papaya, chunked
½ cup cucumber, cubed
1 cup kale, trimmed and chopped
½ cup coconut water

Procedure

1. Combine all the ingredients in a blender and mix until you achieve a smooth consistency.

Serves: 1

Calories: 245 per serving

Pink Panther Medley

You'll love this tasty smoothie even if you're not a fan of the color pink.

Ingredients

1 cup pink grapefruit, peeled, seeds removed, and chunked
½ cup pineapple chunkes
½ cup strawberries, frozen
½ cup non-fat yogurt
¼ cup water

Procedure

1. Combine all the ingredients in a blender and mix until you achieve a smooth consistency.

Serves: 1

Calories: 159 per serving

Green Tea and Veggie Shake

Enjoy this shake loaded with bioactive substances that burns calories.

Ingredients

½ cup broccoli florets
½ cup cauliflower florets
¾ cup green tea
1 cup pineapple chunks

Procedure

1. Combine all the ingredients in a blender and mix until you achieve a smooth consistency.

Serves: 1

Calories: 68 per serving

Fruit n' Nut Shake

A shake recipe that will fill you up without consuming too much calories.

Ingredients

2 pcs. peaches, pitted, peeled and sliced
6 pcs. unsalted almonds

1 cup non-fat yogurt
½ cup almond milk
1 tbsp. flax seeds
Procedure

1. Combine all the ingredients in a blender and mix until you achieve a smooth consistency.

Serves: 1

Calories: 195 per serving

Chapter 4: Metabolism Boosting Main Dishes

Salmon and Roasted Radish

A healthy plate perfect for weight loss dieters like you.

Ingredients

2 pcs. salmon fillets with the skin on
9 pcs. radishes, cut in half
4 pcs. shallots, cut in half
½ tsp. thyme
½ tsp. rosemary
½ tbsp. fresh basil leaf
1 orange
½ tbsp. olive oil
salt and pepper to taste
cooking spray

Procedure

1. Set oven at 425F

2. Lay aluminum foil on a baking tray and coat with cooking spray. Transfer the radish and shallot halves in the tray and drizzle with olive oil. Season with salt and pepper. Toss to coat vegetables well with oil.

3. Sprinkle with rosemary and thyme and place in the oven to cook for 12 minutes. (Remember to stir once)

4. After cooking the vegetables, push them at the sides of the tray and place the tuna fillets with the skin side down at the center. Season again with salt and

pepper. Cut 4 thin slices from the orange and cover the salmon fillets with 2 slices each.

5. Return the tray in the oven to cook for 15 minutes.

6. Meanwhile, take the zest from the orange and set aside.

7. When the fillets are cooked, remove from the tray and throw away the orange slices.

8. Transfer the salmon in a serving plate and squeeze juice from half an orange on top.

9. Take the radish and shallot from the tray and place them in a bowl. Mix with the orange zest and basil leaf. Toss and serve alongside the fish fillets.

Serves: 2

Calories: 244 per serving

Cauli and Curry

Sweet and spicy—this is a flavor-rich dish also dense with nutrients that are good for the body.

Ingredients

2 cups cauliflower florets
1 tsp. curry powder
1 cup coconut milk
1 tsp. garlic, minced
salt and pepper to taste

½ tsp. red pepper flakes
1 tsp. olive oil
½ tsp. cilantro, chopped
Procedure

1. Set oven at 375F.

2. Drizzle the olive oil in a non-stick skillet and heat over medium-low fire. When the pan is hot, sauté the garlic for about a minute.

3. Turn of the heat and combine all the ingredients in an oven-safe dish.

4. Place in the oven to cook for about 30 minutes. Sprinkle with cilantro on top.

Serves: 3

Calories: 190 per serving

Spiced Shrimps

A spiced recipe of shrimp perfect if paired with a green salad.

Ingredients

12 oz. shrimp, peeled and patted dry
2 scallions, chopped
1 bell pepper, chopped
1 tsp. garlic powder
1 tsp. paprika
1 tbsp. olive oil
1 tbsp. safflower oil
salt and pepper to taste

Procedure

1. Heat a non-stick pan over medium-high fire. Drizzle with olive oil and toss the bell pepper in the pan to cook for 4-5 minutes. Stir frequently to evenly cook the peppers. Transfer on a plate and set aside.

2. Meanwhile, coat the shrimps with safflower oil, season with salt, pepper, garlic powder, and paprika. Place them in the pan to cook for 2-4 minutes or until the shrimp's center is opaque.

3. Turn of the heat and add the cooked bell pepper and chopped scallions.

4. Serve with green salad on the side.

Serves: 2

Calories: 144 per serving

Pan-Cooked Citrus Chicken and Mustard Greens

A perfect pairing of chicken and greens that are great fat-burning foods.

Ingredients

2 chicken breast fillets, skin removed
4 cups mustard greens, chopped
¼ cup orange juice
½ orange, peel and seeds removed, chunked
1 cup cooked quinoa

1 tbsp. Dijon mustard
½ tbsp. low-sodium soy sauce
salt and pepper to taste
cooking spray

Procedure

1. Place the mustard seeds in a small bowl and pour the orange juice with it. Set aside.

2. Coat a non-stick pan with cooking spray and heat over medium-high fire. Season the chicken fillets with salt and pepper and cook in the pan for 2-3 minutes each side. Transfer on a plate and set aside.

3. Place the mustard greens in the same skillet and cook for 4 minutes or until the greens wilt. Add the cooked quinoa and orange chunks in the pan with the greens and cook for another 2-3 minutes.

4. Scoop the cooked greens on 2 separate plates.

5. Still using the same pan, pour the orange juice and mustard seed mixture and combine with the Dijon mustard and low-sodium soy sauce. Cook for a few minutes, bringing it to a simmer.

6. Add the chicken fillets to the pan and cook until the chicken is tender.

7. Serve the chicken on top of the mustard greens on the plate and glaze with the orange and mustard seed sauce.

Serves: 2

Calories: 241 per serving

Easy Eggplant Rolls

A hearty dinner using negative calorie foods.

Ingredients

1 medium-sized eggplant, cut into ¼ inch lengthwise
1 ½ cup baby spinach
½ cup fresh basil leaves
2 cups tomatoes, crushed
½ cup red bell peppers, diced
¼ cup white onion, chopped
1 ½ tbsp. garlic, chopped
2 tsp. red pepper flakes
salt to taste
¼ cup toasted almonds, (soak in water for at least 12 hours)
2 tbsp. parmesan cheese, grated
1 tbsp. olive oil
cooking spray

Procedure

1. Set oven at 350F.

2. Coat a non-stick, oven-safe pan with cooking spray and heat over medium-high fire. Throw in the bell pepper and onion and sauté for 4-5 minutes.

3. Add the spinach to the pan and cook for a few minutes until it is wilted. Transfer into a bowl and set aside.

4. Coat the pan again with cooking spray and sauté the garlic for 2-3 minutes. Add the red pepper flakes, basil leaves and stir until the basil leaves wilts.

5. Throw the tomatoes in the pan and continue cooking for 4-5 minutes or until you achieve a thick sauce.

6. Drizzle the eggplant slices with olive oil and season well with salt. Heat the grill and roast the eggplants for a minute on each side.

7. Meanwhile, add ½ of the tomato sauce with the spinach in the bowl and mix well. Season with red pepper flakes again and stir well.

8. Place a cling wrap on top of your kitchen counter and lay the grilled eggplant slices on top. Scoop about 1-22 tbsp. of the spinach mixture on top of the eggplant and carefully roll.

9. Transfer the eggplant rolls in the pan with ½ of the tomato sauce and spoon some of the sauce on top of the eggplant.

10. Place the pan in the oven to cook for 10 minutes, or until the eggplant is tender.

11. While waiting for the eggplants to bake, place the soaked almonds and chop them in the food processor or blender for about a minute until you achieve a thick mixture. Transfer in a small bowl and combine with the parmesan and a pinch of salt.

12. Scoop the almond mixture on two plates and then top with the eggplant roll.

Serves: 2

Calories: 227 per serving

Crab and Greens Salad Plate

An age-old recipe that's perfect for weightwatchers like you!

Ingredients

8 oz. crab meat, cooked and shredded
1 head lettuce, shredded
1 ripe avocado, pitted and chopped
1 small carrot, julienned
1 large tomato, chopped
½ fennel bulb, sliced thin
2 pcs. hard-boiled eggs, sliced

For the dressing:
½ cup zero-fat Greek yogurt
¼ cup plain almond milk
2 tbsp. Sriracha sauce
1 tbsp. grated onion
1 clove of garlic, minced
1 tbsp. parsley, chopped
pinch of cayenne
Salt to taste

Procedure

1. Place all the ingredients of the dressing in a small bowl and whisk well. Set aside.

2. Place the shredded lettuce in a salad bowl and top with tomatoes, carrots, fennel, avocado, crabmeat, and hard-boiled eggs.

3. Serve the salad with the dressing on the side.

Serves: 2

Calories: 246 per serving

Baked Crunchy Fish Fillet

Try this healthier approach to cooking your favorite fish fillet.

Ingredients

2 pcs. halibut fillets (4 oz. each)
½ cup almond flakes
1 egg white, beat lightly
1 tbsp. olive oil
1 pc. lemon, cut into wedges
salt and pepper to taste

Procedure

1. Set the oven at 350F

2. Generously season the fillets with salt and pepper and then brush both sides with lightly beaten egg whites.

3. Place the almond flakes on a plate and carefully coat the seasoned fillets with almond the flakes, making sure that the fish is covered.

4. Drizzle olive oil over an oven-safe, non-stick skillet and transfer the fillets in it. Place the skillet inside the preheated oven to cook until the almonds have turned golden brown.

5. Serve with lemon wedges on the side. This recipe is best eaten with a leafy green salad for a well-rounded meal.

Serves: 2

Calories: 164 per serving

Classic Baked Chicken with Warm Apple and Cabbage Slaw

This is another delicious and ultra-healthy recipe even beginners in the kitchen would find easy to do.

Ingredients

2 4 oz. chicken breast fillet, skin and bone removed
1 small white onion, sliced thin
½ tsp. fennel seeds
1 cup grated apple
4 cups shredded cabbage
1 tbsp. apple cider vinegar
1 tbsp. maple syrup
salt and pepper to taste
1 tbsp. olive oil

Procedure

1. Set the oven at 350F

2. Cut the chicken into strips and generously season with salt and pepper.

3. Heat the olive oil in an oven-safe skillet over medium-high fire. When the oil is hot, place the chicken in the pan and cook for about 2 minutes on

each side, or until they are almost cooked. Transfer on a plate and set aside.

4. Place the sliced onions in the same pan and cook for 2 minutes. Add the fennel seeds, shredded cabbage, and apple.

5. Cover, turn off the heat and transfer the pan in the oven to cook for 8 minutes or until the cabbage and apples are tender.

6. Remove the pan from the oven (do not turn off just yet) and then mix in the apple cider maple syrup. Stir well and season with salt and pepper.

7. Place the chicken on top of the slaw and place in the oven again to cook for 2 minutes.

8. Serve warm.

Serves: 2

Calories: 230 per serving

Vegetarian Stir-fry

Here's a tasty stir-fry recipe loaded with negative calorie ingredients.

Ingredients

3 cups bok choy, chopped
2 cup shiitake mushroom, sliced thin
1 cup bean sprout
½ cup bell pepper, sliced thin
2 cloves of garlic, chopped
1 tsp. ginger, chopped
1 ½ tbsp. coconut aminos, or light soy

2 tsp. green onions, chopped
salt and pepper to taste
1 tbsp. olive oil (divided)

Procedure

1. Heat ½ of the olive oil in a non-stick pan over medium-high fire. Throw in the bean sprouts and stir for about a minute. Remove from the pan and transfer into two separate medium-sized bowls.

2. Drizzle the pan again with the olive oil and heat on medium-high fire. Add the chopped bok choy and bell pepper and stir-fry for about 2-3 minutes or until the bell pepper is tender.

3. Throw in the shiitake to the pan and stir again for 1-2 minutes. Add the garlic and ginger to the pan and continue cooking for 20-30 seconds.

4. Drizzle the coconut aminos to the vegetables and toss to coat. Season with salt and pepper, stir, and turn off heat.

5. Transfer the vegetables on top of the bowls with bean sprouts and garnish with chopped green onions. Serve warm.

Serves: 2

Calories: 97 per serving

Seared Shrimps on Green Pea Purée

Shrimp lovers will fall in love with this hearty recipe.

Ingredients

8 oz. shrimps, skinned and deveined
1 ½ cup green peas
½ cup light coconut milk
1 pc. shallot, sliced thin
½ tsp. thyme
salt to taste
2 tbsp. olive oil (divided)
4 tsp. olive oil
½ tsp. lemon juice
1 tsp. apple cider vinegar
½ tsp. mint leaves, minced
¼ tsp. raw honey

Procedure

1. Drizzle 1 tbsp. olive oil on a non-stick skillet and heat over medium-low fire.

2. Add the shallots, season with a pinch of salt and stir. Cook until the shallots turn light brown.

3. Add the peas, coconut milk, and thyme to the pan. Turn up the heat to medium and cook for about 5 minutes. Transfer the mixture into a blender and purée until smooth. You can add more milk if necessary. Set aside.

4. Heat the remaining 1 tbsp. olive oil on another pan over medium-high fire. Throw in the shrimps and sear until they turn pink. Transfer into a plate and set aside.

5. In a bowl, stir the 4 tsp. olive oil, lemon juice, apple cider, mint leaves, and honey. Season with salt and whisk well.

6. Scoop the green pea purée on a serving plate, top with the seared shrimps and drizzle with the vinaigrette dressing.

7. Serve warm.

Serves: 2

Calories: 259 per serving

Chicken and Veggie Stir-Fry

A simple and easy stir-fry dish that's loaded with negative calorie ingredients. This is a perfect recipe when you don't want to spend too much time in the kitchen.

Ingredients

2 pcs. chicken breast, pre-broiled
3 cloves of garlic
1 small white onion, chopped
½ cup celery, chopped
1 bunch asparagus, cut into bite sized pieces
1 large tomato, chopped
1 tbsp. olive oil
1/8 tsp. flax seed oil
2 tsp. coconut aminos

Procedure

1. Heat the olive and flax seed oil in a wok over medium-high fire.

2. Add the chopped garlic and sauté for about a minute. Add the onions, celery, asparagus, and tomatoes to the pan and stir well.

3. Chop the broiled chicken and add to the pan with the veggies.

4. Stir fry for about 2-4 minutes and then drizzle with coconut aminos.

5. Serve warm.

Serves: 2

Calories: 216 per serving

Greek Salad Bowl

Enjoy the flavors of Greece with this low-calorie, antioxidant packed salad that you can prepare in just 15 minutes!

Ingredients

1 pc. whole-wheat pita bread
1 can garbanzo beans, rinsed and drained
1 large tomato, seeds removed and chopped
1 small cucumber, chopped
¼ cup red onion, chopped
2 tbsp. parsley leaves, chopped
1 tbsp. extra virgin olive oil
2 tbsp. fresh lemon juice
salt and pepper to taste
1 oz. low-fat feta, crumbled

Procedure

1. Slice the pita bread into bite sizes and place in the oven to toast until crispy for about 10 minutes.

2. In a salad bowl, whisk together the olive oil, lemon juice, salt and pepper. Throw in the bowl the garbanzo beans, tomatoes, cucumber, red onion, and parsley. Toss gently making sure that the ingredients are well-coated with the dressing.

3. Serve with the feta crumbles and pita crisps on top.

Serves: 2

Calories: 280 per serving

Moroccan Fish and Veggie Bowl

A classic dish from Morocco, this vegetable loaded bowl combines plenty of negative calorie ingredients to help you burn fat while you eat.

Ingredients

8 oz. tilapia fillet cut into cubes
2 cups sweet potato, diced
1 cup cabbage, chopped
2 cups zucchini, diced
1 pc. carrot, diced
1 pc. turnip, diced
½ cup bell pepper, chopped
½ cup green beans, sliced into bite sized pieces
½ cup garbanzo beans, rinsed and drained
4 tbsp. raisins
2 cloves of garlic, minced
½ cup fresh cilantro leaves, chopped
½ tbsp. Moroccan spice blend
salt to taste
1 tsp. Sriracha sauce
1 tbsp. olive oil

1 cup whole-wheat couscous

Procedure

1. Heat the olive oil in a large pot over medium fire. Add the garlic and Moroccan spice blend and sauté for a minute.

2. Add the sweet potato, cabbage, zucchini, turnip, and carrots and then add water just enough to cover the veggies. Cook on low for 30 minutes or until the veggies are tender.

3. Add the green beans and Sriracha sauce to the pot and season with salt. Simmer for another 12-15 minutes.

4. Scoop the cooked veggies into a blender and purée until smooth.

5. Transfer the purée back to the pot. Add the garbanzos and raisins. Place the fish on top (do not stir) and cover. Cook for about 12-15 minutes.

6. Cook the couscous with boiling water while waiting for the fish to cook. When the couscous is cooked, set aside for about five minutes before fluffing it with a fork.

7. Scoop the fluffed couscous evenly on 2-3 separate serving bowls. Add the cooked veggies and fish on top and garnish with chopped cilantro on top.

Serves: 2-3

Calories: 260 per serving

Turkey Tacos

A healthier approach to a Mexican food favorite.

Ingredients

6 pcs. medium-sized whole-wheat tortillas
12 oz. ground lean turkey
1 small can black beans, rinsed and drained
1 cup lettuce, chopped
½ cup all-natural or low-sodium salsa
1 tbsp. olive oil
salt and pepper to taste

Procedure

1. Place the tortillas on a baking sheet and toast in a hot oven for about 12-15 minutes. Set aside.

2. Drizzle a non-stick skillet with olive oil and heat over medium-high fire. Add the ground turkey and cook for 5-8 minutes or until slightly brown. Season with salt and pepper and stir.

3. Lay the tortillas on a serving plate and evenly distribute the turkey, black beans, lettuce, and salsa.

4. Serve warm.

Serves: 3

Calories: 276 per serving

Sirloin Dinner with Zucchini-Squash Side

This recipes is a good mix protein and veggies for a healthy, well-rounded meal.

Ingredients

2 pcs. 4 oz. sirloin steak, sliced ¾ inch thick
½ tsp. chili powder
¼ tsp. garlic powder
¼ tsp. onion powder
salt and pepper to taste
1 tbsp. olive oil (divided)
¼ cup onion, chopped
1 small zucchini, cut into cubes
2 cups squash, cut into cubes

For the steak sauce:
¼ cup tomato, diced
½ tsp. balsamic vinegar
1 tsp. Worcestershire sauce
¼ cup water
pinch of red pepper flakes
1 tsp. extra virgin olive oil

Procedure

1. Mix the chili, garlic, onion, and a pinch of salt and pepper in a bowl. Season both sides of the steak with the mixture and allow to sit for 10 minutes.

2. Drizzle half of the olive oil on a non-stick pan over medium-hire fire. Throw in the onion, chopped zucchini, and squash to the pan, stir and for 3 minutes or until the veggies are tender. Season with

salt and transfer into a container, cover, and set aside.

3. Heat the remaining oil on the same pan over medium-high fire. Place the steak and cook for 4-5 minutes on each side.

4. While waiting for the steak, mix all the ingredients for the sauce in the bowl except the extra virgin olive oil. Set aside.

5. When cooked, transfer the steak in a cutting board.

6. While heated on medium-high fire, pour the steak sauce to the same pan used to cook the steak and allow to simmer for 3 minutes. Turn off the heat and drizzle with the extra virgin olive oil.

7. Serve the steak with sauce on top and cooked veggies on the side.

Serves: 2

Calories: 235 per serving

Stuffed Bell Pepper Cups

A south-of-the-border recipe that makes use of a variety of negative calorie ingredients.

Ingredients

2 large green bell peppers, top and core removed
½ cup brown rice, cooked
½ cup red beans, rinsed and drained
¼ cup corn kernels

1 small zucchini, diced
½ cup tomatoes, diced
¼ cup fresh cilantro leaves, chopped
1 tbsp. white onion, chopped
1 clove of garlic, minced
pinch of chili powder
salt and pepper to taste
1 tsp. and 1 tbsp. olive oil
4 tbsp. low-fat cheddar cheese, shredded
1 tbsp. low-fat sour cream

Procedure

1. Set oven at 375F.

2. In a bowl, combine the cooked brown rice, beans, corn kernels, zucchini, tomatoes, cilantro, onion, and garlic. Season with chili powder, salt and pepper. Drizzle with 1 tsp. olive oil and mix well.

3. Scoop the mixture evenly, filling up to ¾ of the bell pepper cups.

4. Place the stuffed bell peppers on an oil coated oven-safe pan. Cover the pan with foil and place in the oven to cook for 40 minutes.

5. Remove the foil and top the bell peppers with shredded cheddar. Place back in the oven to melt the cheese for 10 minutes.

6. Serve the bell peppers with a scoop of sour cream.

Serves: 2

Calories: 242 per serving

Conclusion

Thank you again for purchasing this book! I hope it changed your perspective that going on a diet and losing weight isn't synonymous with hunger and food deprivation.

Remember, that as long as you pick the right foods that help burn fat and choose whole foods that are nutritious, (plus of course, regular exercise) you can achieve your health goals such as shedding weight and boosting your metabolism. It only takes 30 days for you to see the benefits of eating healthy, and after the diet, your lifestyle will also change because you will be wiser in choosing the foods you eat.

I hope that you try the recipes I shared with you in this book and also, don't be afraid to try and make your own Negative Calorie Diet recipes!

Made in the USA
Lexington, KY
21 June 2016